POWER DRESSING
MEN'S FASHION AND PRESTIGE IN AFRICA

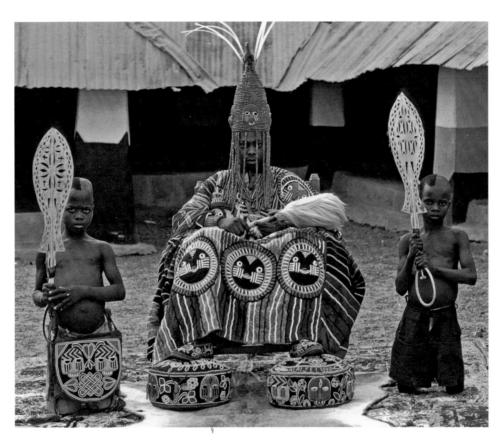

THE NEWARK MUSEUM

Published in conjunction with the exhibition
Power Dressing: Men's Fashion and Prestige in Africa

The Newark Museum, Newark, New Jersey
October 19, 2005 – January 22, 2006

Parrish Art Museum, Southampton, New York
April 2 – May 28, 2006

Power Dressing: Men's Fashion and Prestige in Africa is made possible by The Coby Foundation, Ltd, the Prudential Foundation, the LINKS of Essex County, and the New Jersey Council for the Humanities

The Newark Museum, a not-for-profit museum of art, science and education, receives operating support from the City of Newark, the State of New Jersey, the New Jersey State Council on the Arts/Department of State (a Partner Agency of the National Endowment for the Arts) and corporate, foundation and individual donors. Funds for acquisitions and activities other than operations are provided by members and other contributors.

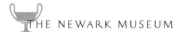

THE NEWARK MUSEUM

49 Washington Street
Newark, New Jersey 07102-3176
www.NewarkMuseum.org

Design: Marc Zaref Design, Inc.
Printing: The Studley Press
Photography: Richard Goodbody, with the exception of pl. 7 (Douglas Dawson), pl. 14 (Brooklyn Museum) and pl. 26 (Donald J. Martin)

All photographs in situ by Eliot Elisofon reproduced in this publication were provided by the Eliot Elisofon Photographic Archives (EEPA), National Museum of African Art, Smithsonian Institution.

cover: (detail) Ceremonial robe of the Déjì of Akure, late 19th – early 20th century, Akure, Ekiti region, Nigeria; Yoruba, cotton, velvet, beads; 50 x 104 ½ in. The Newark Museum, Purchase 1993 John J. O'Neil Bequest Fund & The Member's Fund, 93.268

title page: Oba Ademuwagun Adesida II, the Déjì of Akure, on throne in courtyard of Akure palace, Yoruba peoples, Nigeria, Photograph by Eliot Elisofon, 1959 (EEPA no. 2071)

back cover: (detail) Tunic, ca. 1990s (back), Djenne, Mali; Bozo or Fulani, cotton, embroidery floss; 45 x 25 in., The Newark Museum, Gift of Joseph Knopfelmacher 1997, 97.22.1

FOREWORD

Museums are called upon to mount exhibitions that showcase unique collections, and in that regard, *Power Dressing: Men's Fashion and Prestige in Africa* is a superb example. The Newark Museum, groundbreaking in so many collecting areas, has a long-established interest in African art, and particularly in African textiles. The Museum began collecting textiles from northern Africa and sub-Saharan Africa in the 1920s, and seven works in this exhibition date to that early period. In more recent decades, former curator Anne M. Spencer, together with my predecessor, Samuel C. Miller, made many inspired acquisitions of African cloth, culminating in the national touring exhibition—jointly organized with the UCLA Fowler Museum of Cultural History—*Wrapped in Pride: Ghanaian Kente and African American Identity*.

In *Power Dressing*, Dr. Christa Clarke, The Newark Museum's Curator of Africa, the Americas and the Pacific, examines an important and, until now, neglected aspect of African dress. She mines the rich heritage of men's attire in Africa for its symbolic as well as aesthetic significance; the result of her scholarship is the first American museum exhibition to examine this topic. We are particularly proud of her work, and proud as well that so many of the ensembles are drawn from the Museum's own collections. They are complemented by other important art works generously lent by both public and private collectors.

Power Dressing has also provided the impetus for The Newark Museum to reach out to members of New Jersey's growing African diasporic community. The Trustees and staff are deeply grateful to the Honorable Donald M. Payne, Congressman from New Jersey, and the Honorable Barack Obama, Senator from Illinois, for graciously co-chairing the Honorary Committee. They are joined by writer Dr. Chinua Achebe and a host of other distinguished representatives of this community in the Metropolitan area. For her guidance in these matters, I also thank Isimeme Omogbai, The Newark Museum's Chief Operating Officer.

As always, such complicated exhibitions and related public programming would not be possible without the generous support of the Museum's partners, especially the City of Newark, the State of New Jersey, the New Jersey State Council on the Arts/Department of State, The Geraldine R. Dodge Foundation, and the Victoria Foundation. Special funds for *Power Dressing* have been contributed by The Coby Foundation, Ltd., the Prudential Foundation, the LINKS of Essex County, and the New Jersey Council for the Humanities.

The Newark Museum is fortunate to be at the confluence of a rich collection, dedicated patrons and emerging audiences. To those patrons and our new friends, we offer *Power Dressing* as a lively, edifying and educational experience.

Mary Sue Sweeney Price
Director

ACKNOWLEDGMENTS

This exhibition quite literally emerged from the depths of storage, as I began to familiarize myself with the Museum's holdings of African textiles shortly after coming here in 2002. This aspect of the Museum's African collection dates to the early twentieth century, but owes its renown today in part to former curator Anne Spencer, who carefully and creatively developed the collection during her twenty-five-year tenure. I was particularly struck by the exceptional artistry and diversity of the examples of men's prestige attire in our collection. Conversations with colleagues Vicki Rovine and Hélène Joubert helped shape my ideas for a possible exhibition, and I appreciate their enthusiastic responses to the collection. The opportunity to bring these works together as a major exhibition presented itself in the summer of 2004, and I am grateful to many colleagues, lenders, and friends for helping to make this exhibition possible in a short period of time.

Foremost, I would like to acknowledge my deep gratitude to those lenders who have contributed to this exhibition. Many thanks to Arnold Lehman, Bill Siegmann, and Elisa Flynn at The Brooklyn Museum, and to Howard C. Collinson and Donald J. Martin at The University of Iowa Museum of Art for facilitating important loans from their respective institutions. Drs. Marian and Daniel Malcolm and Dr. and Mrs. Bernard Wagner generously agreed to part with treasured works from their collections, as did Gary van Wyk and Lisa Brittan of Axis Gallery in New York. I am also grateful to Holly and David Ross for granting me access to their collection and for their contributions toward this exhibition.

Many individuals aided in the research phase, graciously sharing information, ideas, and assistance. I would like to thank Shuaib Ahmed (New Jersey), Kathleen Bickford Berzock (Art Institute of Chicago), Suzanne Blier (Harvard University), Alban Bronsin (Brussels, Belgium), Lisa Brittan (Axis Gallery), Amadou Diallo (New Jersey), Henry Drewal (University of Wisconsin), Silvia Forni (Universitadi Torino, Italy), Bernhard Gardi (Museum der Kulturen, Basel), Christraud Geary (Museum of Fine Arts, Boston), Father Hermann Gufler (Oku, Cameroon), Hélène Joubert (Musée Quai Branly, Paris), Colleen Kriger (University of North Carolina at Greensboro), Clement Alexander Price (Rutgers University, Newark), Doran Ross (Los Angeles), Victoria Rovine (University of Florida, Gainesville), Bill Siegmann (Brooklyn Museum), Anne Spencer (New Jersey), Amy Staples (Eliot Elisofon Photographic Archives, National Museum of African Art, Smithsonian Institution), and Gary van Wyk (Axis Gallery). I am especially grateful to my good friend and colleague Kathleen Bickford Berzock for her careful review of and thoughtful comments on my essay.

At The Newark Museum, the collective talents of many staff members contributed to the realization of the exhibition. The daunting challenge of researching many works in a short time was ably met by Harriet Walker, research assistant in the Department of Africa, the Americas, and the Pacific, who also prepared the extensive bibliography, librarian William Peniston, who responded to many requests promptly and cheerfully, and intern Sarah Burford. Millicent Matthews helped in numerous important ways as did Erica Stephen, Mary Dowd, and Bertha Freeman. In the Registrar's Office, I would like to thank Rebecca Buck, Amber Germano, Batja Bell, and especially Scott Hankins, who coordinated loan arrangements and helped prepare our works for exhibition. Exhibition designer Rick Randall has once again worked his magic in developing an innovative exhibition design, with conservator Linda Niewenhuizen, mount-maker Mark Nolden and preparator Bari Falese contributing to their beautiful presentation. The outstanding array of educational and collaborative programs organized in connection with *Power Dressing* represents the creativity and hard work of our education department, led by Lucy Voorhees Brotman, and staff members Linda Nettleton, Sheila Anderson, and Kim Robledo-Diga. The exhibition and its programs will reach a wide audience through the direction provided by our Deputy Director for Marketing and Public Relations, Mark Albin, and his staff, especially the exceptional efforts of Public Relations Manager Lorraine McConnell, and of Community Relations Advisor Ugonma Achebe, who is reaching out to regional audiences of the contemporary African diaspora. Zette Emmons, the Museum's Manager of Traveling Exhibitions has ensured that the exhibition will reach an even wider audience through its other venues.

This beautiful catalogue is the product of the artistic eye and skills of designer Marc Zaref of Marc Zaref Design, Inc. The Museum's Marketing Communications Manager, U. Michael Schumacher, supervised its production with his usual good sense and good humor. Many thanks also to Deputy Director for Development, Peggy Dougherty, and her staff for identifying funders within a compressed time frame. I am especially grateful to have the support of The Coby Foundation and its Director, Ward Mintz, who provided funds for the catalogue. For their staunch support of this exhibition since its inception and unfailing advocacy on its behalf, I extend my deep appreciation to Senior Curator Valrae Reynolds and especially to Chief Operating Officer Isimeme Omogbai, who opened doors to local Nigerian communities and who herself supremely embodies the ongoing relevance of African fashion. Most importantly, I would like to thank Mary Sue Sweeney Price, who has enthusiastically encouraged the development of this exhibition, for her forward-thinking vision as Director and ongoing commitment to presenting the artistry of the African continent at The Newark Museum.

Christa Clarke
Curator of Africa, the Americas and the Pacific

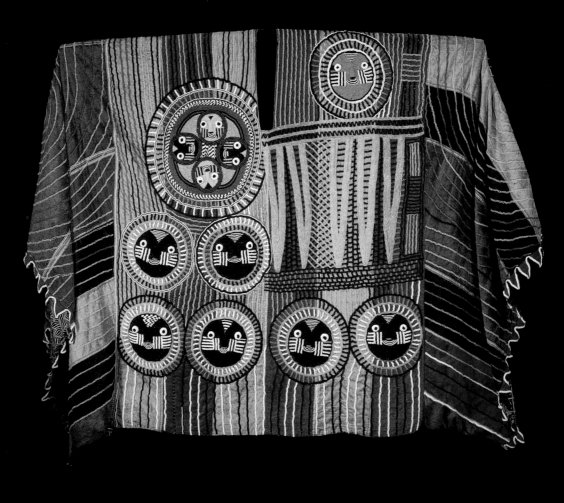

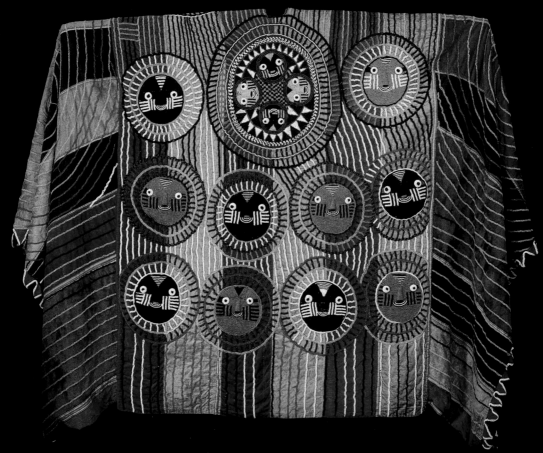

POWER DRESSING: MEN'S FASHION AND PRESTIGE IN AFRICA

Christa Clarke

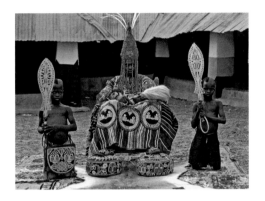

On November 19, 1959, Oba Ademuwagan Adesida II posed in the courtyard of his palace for *Life* magazine photographer Eliot Elisofon. Nigeria's first federal election was just one month away, and the country was headed for independence after almost seven decades of British colonial rule. At the time, Oba Adesida II was a 34-year-old regional leader, or Déjì, of the Yoruba, one of the largest ethnic groups in Nigeria, ruling Akure as the 42nd Déjì to hold that elevated post. This Déjì was also an attorney who had studied law in Dublin and passed the bar examination in London. In Akure, where his authority extended over more than 100,000 people, the Déjì was striving to introduce electricity and piped water into the city. Reflecting on the ruler's position within this changing political and social landscape, photographer Elisofon described the Déjì as a "young European-educated leader who holds a tradition-encrusted throne, and is attempting to reconcile the two cross-currents...The Déjì, in one man, embodies much of the contrast between old and new that is so striking throughout Nigeria, and it is partly because of this that he is a fascinating man."[1]

In the photograph, the Déjì poses in ceremonial regalia, flanked by two young attendants bearing ceremonial swords. The Déjì's choice of dress is significant, for it was intended to emphasize the power and authority of traditional systems of leadership in a rapidly changing Nigeria. On his head, the Déjì wears a tall, beaded crown with a veil that obscures his face, underscoring his sacred nature. His feet, in elaborately beaded slippers, are supported by beaded foot cushions placed on a lion skin rug. In his hands, he holds a beaded whisk.

A particularly important element in the Déjì's public presentation is his beaded robe (pl. 1; cat. 1), a "wonderfully hybrid garment" that has been the subject of close analysis by art historian Henry Drewal.[2] In style, the robe is a Yoruba version of the Hausa "robe of honor" worn by the political elite to the north. The Déjì's robe is made of velvet, a luxury import that emphasizes the ruler's privileged access to foreign goods. The velvet has been cut into strips and sewn together in imitation of a type of high-status Yoruba cloth known as *aso-oke*. Extensive beadwork covers the garment. According to Yoruba belief, embellishment with beads, symbolic of royalty, increases the ritual potency of the regalia.

1

Ceremonial robe of the Déjì of Akure (front and back), late 19th – early 20th century
Akure, Ekiti region, Nigeria; Yoruba
Cotton, velvet, beads; 50 x 104 ½ in.

The Newark Museum, Purchase 1993 John J. O'Neil Bequest Fund & The Member's Fund, 93.268

The beadwork designs reflect both tradition and change. Small beadwork faces representing the original Yoruba kings situate the Déjì within the royal lineage as a sacred descendant of Oduduwa, a Yoruba god and their first ruler. At the same time, Hausa designs have been adapted or replaced with Yoruba icons of power. On the Déjì's left, elongated triangles are Hausa motifs referred to as "knives" symbolizing wealth. On the right, a large circle with four faces evokes a Yoruba divination board, replacing the spiral design typically embroidered on Hausa robes while retaining its protective symbolism.

The Déjì's robe, with its many layers of meaning, exemplifies the complex issues underlying the relationship between men's dress and power in Africa. Throughout the continent, men generally occupy more visible spaces of power in the social, political, and spiritual realms than do women.[3] Dress is central to a man's self presentation in such contexts, serving as an important marker of power and status.[4] The ceremonial dress and prestige attire of African men are intended to have dramatic visual impact and are designed to impress the viewer with their aesthetic and symbolic power.

Power Dressing: Men's Fashion and Prestige in Africa brings together fifty examples of spectacular male attire spanning the continent from Morocco to South Africa and representing over a century of fashion. The works, which vary tremendously in style, form, material and technique, are drawn primarily from The Newark Museum's own important holdings as well as significant examples from private and public collections. Rather than presenting a geographic or chronological survey, the exhibition explores the artistry of men's dress as it relates to and embodies social, political, and spiritual power. The works are presented in four broad and intersecting themes that provide rich insights into the meanings of men's fashions within Africa's diverse and ever-changing cultural and political landscape.

STYLE AND STATUS

In many ways, dress can be considered a visual language, an aesthetic code expressing ideas about status.[5] Stylistic choices—such as material, texture, color, cut—may send messages about the wearer's status, whether social, economic, political, occupational, religious, or a combination of the above. At once inclusive and exclusive, dress establishes the wearer's membership in a certain group while distinguishing him from others.[6] As such, a man's clothing is an important vehicle through which power may be defined, sustained, negotiated, or reinforced.[7]

In some contexts, a man's status is expressed visually through volume, measured by the amount of material used, its cost, the difficulty of its manufacture, and the extent of decorative embellishment. The hooded cloak (pl. 2; cat. 2), or *akhnif*, once widely worn by Berber men of the Ait Ouaouzguite

2

Cloak (*akhnif*), late 19th – early 20th century
Sus region, Morocco; Ait Ouaouzguite
Wool; 63 x 71 ½ in.

The Newark Museum, Purchase 1927,
The J. Ackerman Coles Collection, 27.105

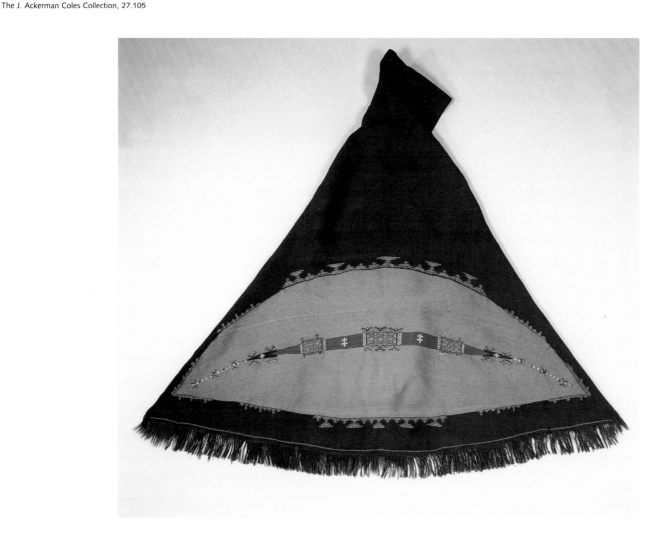

confederation in rural Morocco, represents the skillful and painstaking work of female weavers. This visually spectacular men's garment is prized for its dramatic size and, especially, for its elaborate method of weaving wool into a semicircular shape, a technique seen also in cloaks worn in Coptic Egypt.[8] The long elliptical eye-shaped design on the back of the cloak has been interpreted as a protective symbol intended to ward off the "evil eye."[9]

A major form of men's prestige attire across western Africa is the voluminous tailored, embroidered gown worn bunched at the shoulders, a type of garment known as a *boubou* throughout French-speaking West Africa.[10] Although in sub-Saharan Africa, the wearing of such robes is historically associated with the Islamic faith and lifestyle, the garments are not expressly religious and, in fact, became fashionable in non-Islamic communities. Of the many types of prestige robes found in West Africa, the embroidered gowns worn by Hausa-Fulani men represent a particularly important and influential dress tradition. Hausa-Fulani men's dress played a critical role in maintaining unity and central authority in the Sokoto Caliphate (ca. 1810-1908), a powerful federation of emirates located in what is now northern Nigeria. Expensive tailored gowns with lavish embroidery, called *riga* in the Hausa language, became an integral part of investiture ceremonies and were distributed as gifts to high-ranking officials.[11] These visually stunning "robes of honor" identified the wearer as a member of the Hausa-Fulani ruling class and remained an important means of cultural identity throughout the twentieth century to the present day.

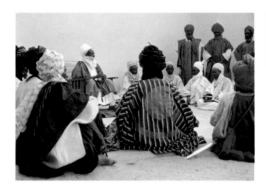

The Emir of Katsina, Morning greeting ceremony, Hausa peoples, Nigeria. Photograph by Eliot Elisofon, 1959 (EEPA no. 1383).

The Hausa *riga* in this exhibition (pl. 3; cat. 3) was made in the late 1920s for a chief or wealthy trader in the Zaria region. The *riga* is of white cotton damask with embroidery in green wool, imported materials that were highly valued and whose use reflects the increased access to trade goods in the early twentieth century as a result of the construction of a railroad from Lagos to the north.[12] The extensive embroidery was done by hand by a *malam*, a male religious specialist with knowledge of Arabic writing.[13] The designs, drawn from an Islamic visual vocabulary international in scope, refer to political leadership and offer protective powers.[14] These motifs include the *tambari* or "king's drum," a spiral motif on the wearer's right chest, signifying Hausa chieftaincy.

The *riga* is part of a larger ensemble worn by an elite man that can include one or more robes as undergarments, embroidered drawstring trousers (cat. 4), a turban, a flowing cloak, leather boots (cat. 5), and, possibly, a prestige staff (cat. 6). The combination of volume and layering creates an overall "aesthetic of bigness" that enhances both the physical presence and symbolic importance of the wearer.[15] The trousers with embroidery (*wando mai surfani*), for example, have a waistline of over fifteen feet and are embellished with multicolored geometric designs. Worn baggy and gathered around the waist, the expansive size of the trousers and elaborate embroidery affirm the wealth of the wearer. A studied disregard for cost is

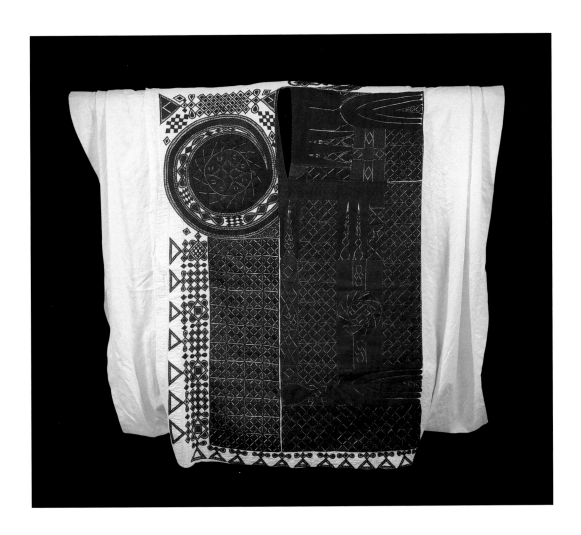

3
Robe (*riga*), 1920s (detail: right)
Zaria, Nigeria; Hausa
Cotton, wool; 57 x 103 in.

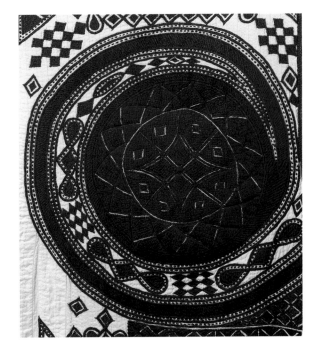

reinforced by the fact that such expensive and striking embellishment would be hidden under a robe, seen only briefly if the wearer was on horseback, representing the ultimate in "inconspicuous consumption."[16]

The Hausa-Fulani style of dress had considerable regional impact through both trade and politics. In the early nineteenth century, the non-Muslim Yoruba to the south adopted and adapted the style, following the conquest of the Yoruba empire of Oyo by the Fulani in the 1830s. The Yoruba *agbada* and its variants convey the wearer's status through subtle distinctions in the type of cloth and its quality, and the garment's cut and workmanship, as well as the style and fashion of embroidery and other ornamentation. For example, the richly embroidered, hand-woven *agbada* of beige raw silk (pl. 4; cat. 7), known as *sanyan*, is among the most expensive and prestigious of robes. The locally produced silk is not cultivated, making it extremely valuable. Such garments continue to be prized by many Yoruba, and are worn especially by the political and religious elite as an expression of respect for the traditions of the past.[17] Since 1999, the wearing of *agbada* by Nigerian president Olusegun Obasanjo and other high-ranking leaders

4

Robe (*agbada*), early 20th century (detail: opposite)
Oyo, Nigeria; Yoruba
Silk, cotton; 49 x 97 in.

The Newark Museum, Purchase 1986 The Member's Fund, 86.240

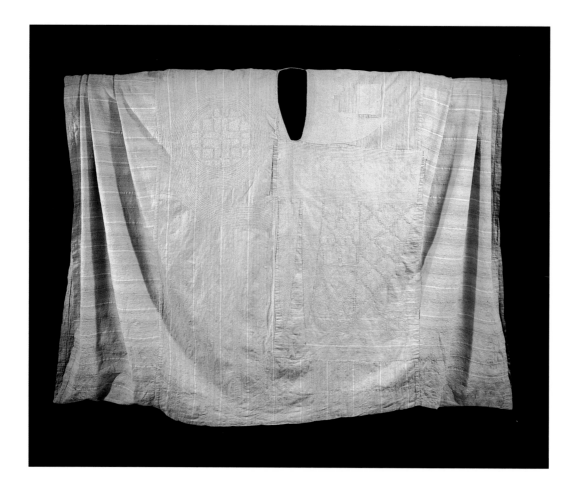

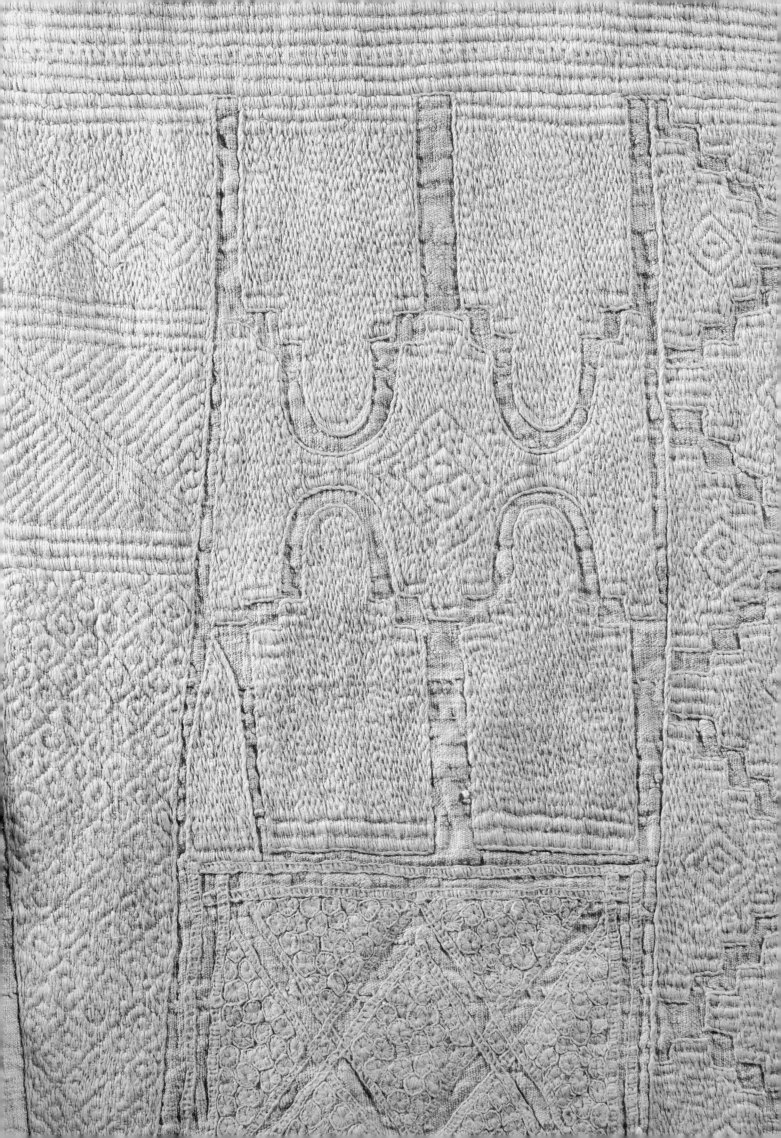

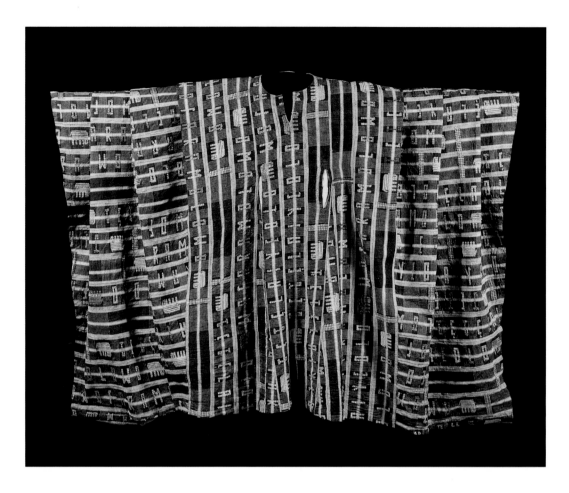

5
Robe (*dandogo*), mid-20th century
Nigeria; Yoruba
Cotton; 46 ½ x 109 in.
The Newark Museum, Purchase 1983 Wallace
M. Scudder Bequest Fund, 83.102

has had political implications at a national level, a strategic choice of dress meant to signify the country's transition to democracy after decades of colonial and postcolonial military rule.[18]

The *dandogo*, a variant of the northern-style robe developed by the Yoruba, is distinguished by two slit-like openings in the front, which originally enabled the wearer to hold the reins of a horse.[19] Reflecting the Yoruba love for novelty in fashion, a strip-woven *dandogo* (pl. 5; cat. 9) features weft patterning in the form of letters interspersed with elephant motifs. The introduction of literary and pictorial motifs as design elements in Yoruba weaving appears to be an innovation dating to the mid- to late twentieth century.[20] The robe's woven text refers to a Yoruba proverb whose meaning may be interpreted as "The world is changeable, but the rich stick together," intended to leave no doubt as to the wearer's comfortable economic position and social status.[21]

In contrast to the "aesthetic of bigness" seen in West African men's robes, minimal clothing may be the norm for men in other African societies. Dinka men in the southern part of Sudan traditionally consider it unmanly to cover the body. As cattle herders whose wanderings have necessitated the portability of their personal possessions, a Dinka man's primary form of clothing was a tightly buttoned corset made of multiple strands of beads. This type of dress developed, in part, as a result of the greater abundance of glass trade beads in the region.[22] Its form is designed to emphasize a slender waist, and its patterning relates to age and wealth. The alternating red and black beads on this example (pl. 6; cat. 10) indicate that the wearer was between 15 and 25 years old, while the height of the projection at back suggests that he came from a family wealthy in cattle. Today, such corsets are often replaced with a simple beaded belt.

Among the Lega, in the Democratic Republic of the Congo, headdresses are the primary means through which men distinguish their status in *bwami*, a graded, socio-political organization open to all

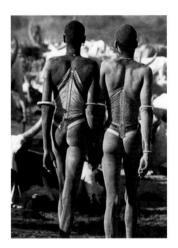

Dinka herders in beaded corsets walk among cattle in their dry season camp, Lake Nybor, Sudan.
Photograph © Carol Beckwith and Angela Fisher, 1981.

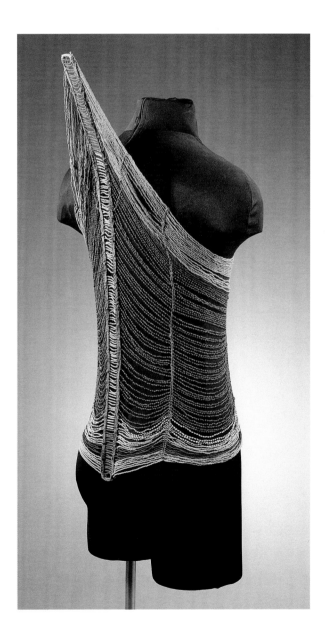

6

Man's corset, second half of the 20th century
Sudan; Dinka
Beads, fiber, leather; 30 x 14 ½ in.

The Newark Museum, Purchase 2005 The Member's Fund, 2005.14

Lega adults. The wearing of certain types of hats is considered an exclusive privilege of high-ranking members and represents their acquired wisdom. Men at the very highest levels of *bwami* wear a type of hat, known as *sawamazembe,* made of braids of plaited fiber and adorned with mussel shells (pl. 7; cat. 11). Its form, an imitation of a female initiate's hairstyle, and material, particularly the polished mussel shell valves adorning the front, symbolize the female power that, in combination with maleness, is necessary for the highest levels of leadership.[23] Hats surmounted by elephant tail and adorned with cowries or beads (*mukuba wa bifungo*), signify that the wearer has just progressed to the highest grade (cat. 12).[24] Those adorned with the skin of a pangolin, an animal associated with family and clan, are worn by men in lower grades who rely on their kin for acceptance and advancement (cat. 13).[25]

7
Headdress (*sawamazembe*), 20th century
Democratic Republic of the Congo; Lega
Fiber, shells, buttons, seed pods; 16¾ x 10 in.
Private Collection

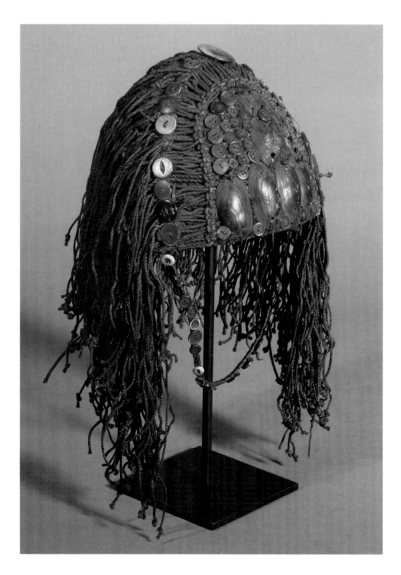

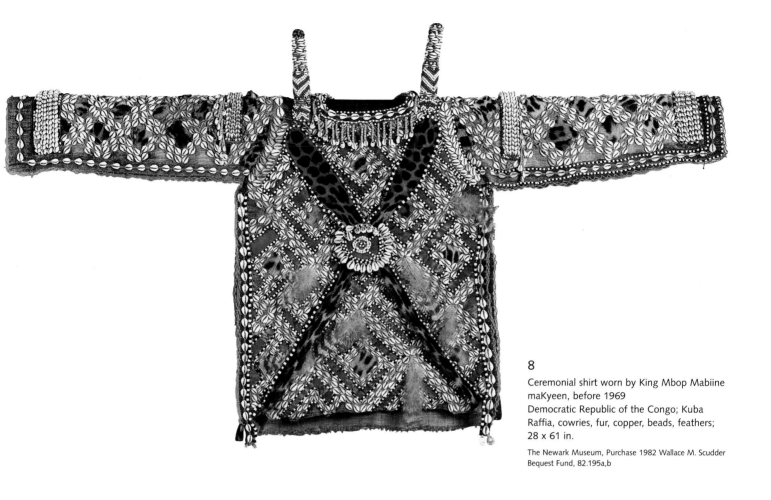

8
Ceremonial shirt worn by King Mbop Mabiine maKyeen, before 1969
Democratic Republic of the Congo; Kuba
Raffia, cowries, fur, copper, beads, feathers; 28 x 61 in.

The Newark Museum, Purchase 1982 Wallace M. Scudder Bequest Fund, 82.195a,b

FIT FOR A KING

The dress of leaders is especially designed for public presentation in formal contexts that establish, enhance or reinforce a ruler's political persona.[26] Leadership dress is by definition exclusive, visually reinforcing a ruler's privileged access through forms, materials, or decorative embellishments restricted to royal use. The power of a leader is emphasized by the sheer size and visual splendor of his ceremonial ensemble, which includes not only clothes but also jewelry, headgear, footwear, and hand-held and other accessories. Usually the form, materials, and designs of a ruler's dress have symbolic meanings related to his wealth, power, and leadership qualities. These meanings are subject to change over time, given the

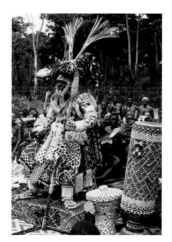

Kuba Nyim (king) Kot aMbweeky III in state dress with royal drum in Mushenge, Zaire (now Democratic Republic of the Congo). Photograph by Eliot Elisofon, 1971 (EEPA no. 2137).

complicated relationship between traditional forms of leadership and colonial and postcolonial government in Africa.

Leadership dress typically reflects the power and wealth of the state rather than expressing an individual's style.[27] The sumptuous ceremonial dress, or *bwaantshy*, of a Kuba king embodies state wealth in its lavish use of cowries, imported glass beads, precious metals, leopard skin, expensive raffia textiles (cat. 14), and other luxury materials. The king's presentation in state dress visually recalls the founding of the dynasty in the seventeenth century and links the present ruler to Woot, the mythical first king. The entire ensemble may consist of nearly fifty objects weighing as much as 185 pounds.[28] The Kuba tunic (pl. 8; cat. 15) and hat presented in this exhibition were part of a larger ceremonial ensemble once owned by the Kuba king Mbop aMabiine maKyeen, who ruled from 1939 to 1969.

In the Akan-speaking kingdoms of Ghana, the royal regalia of a chief or king might easily number over twenty cast-gold or gold-leafed ornaments, including disk pendants (cat. 16 and pl. 9; cat. 17), bracelets (cat. 18), and other jewelry, in addition to gold-accented accessories such as sandals and crowns. Gold was an important source of regional wealth that contributed to the prosperity of Akan kingdoms and particularly to the formation of the Asante state around 1700. The extraordinary quantities of gold regalia displayed on state occasions throughout the Akan kingdoms to this day are both visually dazzling and serve a symbolic function. Regarded as the earthly embodiment of the sun, gold also represented an individual's spiritual essence or *kra*, and by extension, the soul of the Asante nation.

Of primary importance as a symbol of state are the gold-ornamented sandals once worn by an Asante chief (cat. 19). Doran Ross observes that sandals are so closely identified with a ruler in most Akan states that they require the services of a special court official devoted to their security and care.[29] Sandals prevent a ruler's feet from touching the earth, an action considered to have the potential to harm the community. For this reason, they may also be adorned with gold amulets that have a protective function.

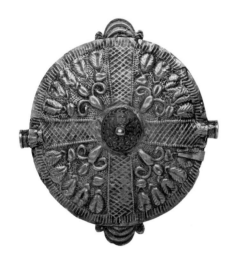

9
Disk pendant (*akrafokonmu*), 20th century
Ghana; Asante
Cast gold; 4 x 4 x 1 in.
The Newark Museum, Purchase 1987 William M. Scudder Bequest Fund, 87.35

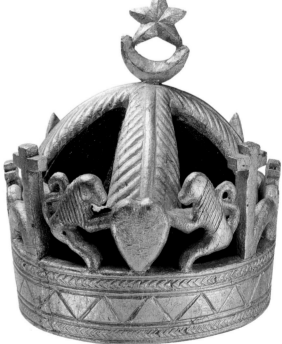

10
Crown, 20th century
Ghana; Asante
Wood, velvet, cotton, gold leaf; 8 ¾ x 8 x 8 in.
The Newark Museum, Purchase 1986 Eleanor S. Upton Bequest Fund, 86.247

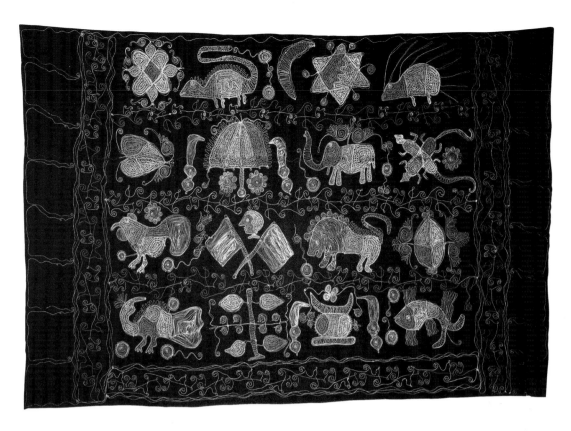

11
"Cloth of the great" (*akunitan*), 1957-66
(detail: overleaf)
Ghana; Akan
Wool, rayon thread; 75 ½ x 115 ½ in.

The Newark Museum, Purchase 2005 The Membership
Endowment Fund, 2005.2

Akan leaders have also adapted certain forms of royal regalia, such as European-style crowns, from the British during the colonial period. Although crowns were a defining emblem of European monarchy, they did not have the same ritual significance among the Akan. The gold leaf and velvet crown (pl. 10; cat. 20) in this exhibition combines symbols related to Akan proverbs, such as the star and moon at top, with designs reflecting the influence of European heraldry, including rampant lions flanking a heart, fleur-de-lis, and crown motifs.[30]

For ceremonial occasions, Akan royal men traditionally wear a voluminous cloth wrapped around the body like a toga, leaving the right shoulder bare. One well-known type is the strip-woven textile called *kente* (cat. 21), made of silk, cotton, or rayon in a dizzying variety of named patterns distinguished by the complexity of their design. Lesser known, perhaps, and of more recent invention is the "cloth of the great," or *akunitan*, which features colorful motifs machine-embroidered on imported British blankets (pl. 11; cat. 22). This type of cloth is worn only by paramount chiefs whose wealth, power, and leadership are alluded to through a variety of representational and abstract symbols. On this cloth are traditional icons of chiefly might, such as a porcupine, elephant, and an umbrella with state swords, combined with a more

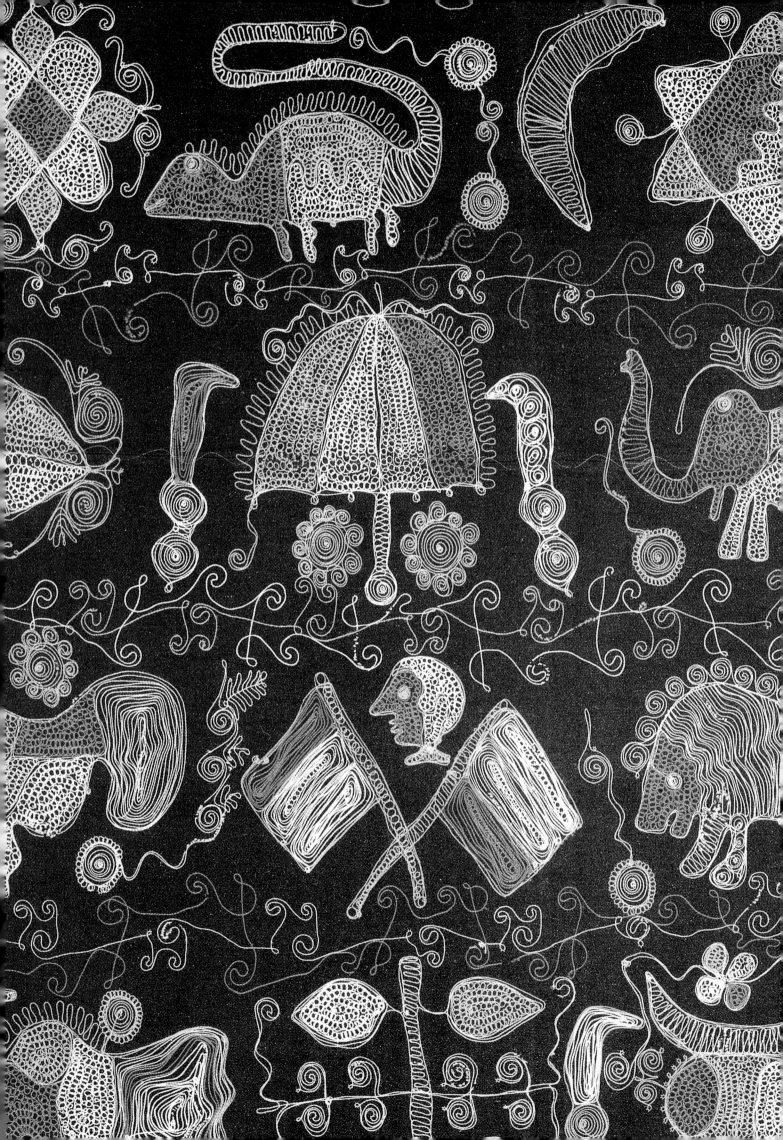

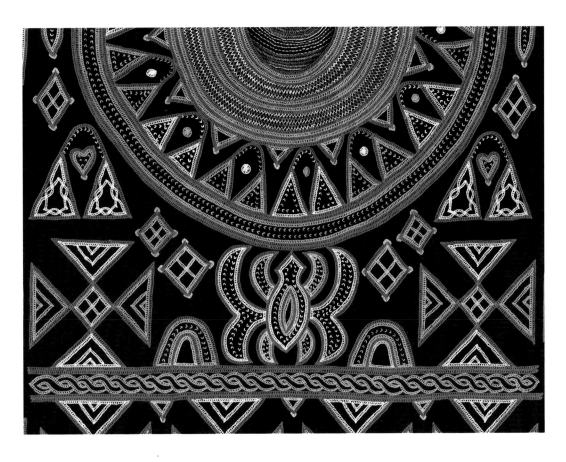

17
Ceremonial gown, 1992 (detail)
Cameroon; Bafut
Polyester, cotton; 50 x 80 ½ in.

The Newark Museum, Purchase 1994 Membership
Endowment Fund, 94.97a

exhibition (pl. 17; cat. 33) has a central motif that combines the forms of two important royal icons—the spider, associated with wisdom and used in divination, and the frog, a symbol of a leader's fertility—as well as other leadership icons such as the double gong. According to Tamara Northern, this deliberate fusion "underpins the visual and contextual discourse of multiple symbols that coherently reinforce each other in the articulation of royal power."[42] The incorporation of such Grassfields-specific designs represents one of the ways that artists adapted a foreign form of dress, introduced by Hausa traders in the nineteenth century, to the tastes of local rulers, known as *fons*. By the turn of the century, a unique type of royal gown evolved in the Western Grassfields, creatively combining cloth and thread imported from Europe with Hausa tailoring and embroidery techniques.[43] The Grassfields gown became a *fon's* preferred dress for diplomacy or other power negotiations beyond the village level during the colonial period and, in recent decades, has increasingly signified cultural unity and traditional values at both regional and national levels.[44]

DIVINE DRESS

Men's dress can relate to spiritual power in multiple and complex ways. The wearing of certain types of clothing or materials may be restricted to religious specialists. The use of symbolic materials, such as beads, or sacred designs, can sanctify dress or allow the wearer to connect with the spiritual realm. While systems of religious belief are expressed through dress in diverse ways, throughout northern and western Africa the influence of Islam has been a particularly strong, and at times unifying, force for dress traditions relating to spirituality.

A type of tunic with stylized appliqué patches known as a *jibbeh* (pl. 18; cat. 36) was worn by high-ranking officers of the Islamic Mahdist army, who fought to liberate Sudan from foreign rule in the late nineteenth century. Led by Sufi holy man Muhammed Ahmed, who proclaimed himself al-Mahdi ("the Divinely Inspired One"), the Mahdis based their military uniforms on the religious dress of Sufi Muslims, whose ragged, patched garments symbolized their ritual poverty. On the tunic of a high-ranking military officer, however, these patches were no longer functional but served as a visual metaphor

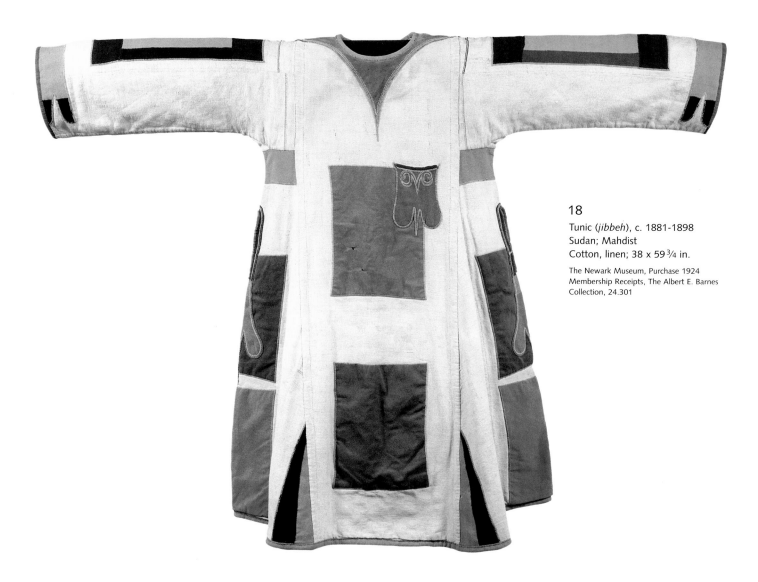

18

Tunic (*jibbeh*), c. 1881-1898
Sudan; Mahdist
Cotton, linen; 38 x 59¾ in.

The Newark Museum, Purchase 1924
Membership Receipts, The Albert E. Barnes
Collection, 24.301

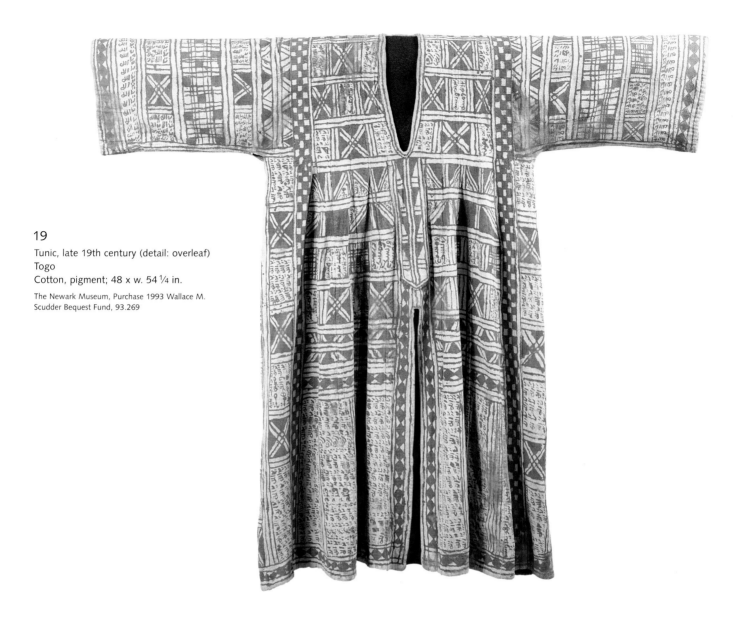

19

Tunic, late 19th century (detail: overleaf)
Togo
Cotton, pigment; 48 x w. 54 ¼ in.

of religious inspiration.[45] At the same time, the stylization and high visibility of the patches reinforced central authority and military rank, in sharp contrast to their conceptual basis in Sufi ideals of equality and communal ownership.[46]

A late nineteenth-century tunic from Togo (pl. 19; cat. 37) literally enveloped the wearer in spirituality, as it is painted with Arabic inscriptions and mystical designs that offer religious protection. It was likely the dress of a man who was a warrior, hunter, or in a similarly dangerous profession and therefore in need of security. The schematized rendering of the word "Allah" that covers the garment provides a visual counterpart to the chanted repetition of Islamic prayers, infusing the textile with the presence of God.[47]

In Mande-speaking societies in Mali and beyond, hunters historically have worn shirts (*donson dlokiw*) that offered spiritual protection from the extraordinary dangers they faced and also marked their exceptional skills and powers.[48] One type of shirt worn by Bamana hunters is made from *bògòlanfini*, a cloth distinguished by the unusual technique of using fermented mud as dye and by its distinctive

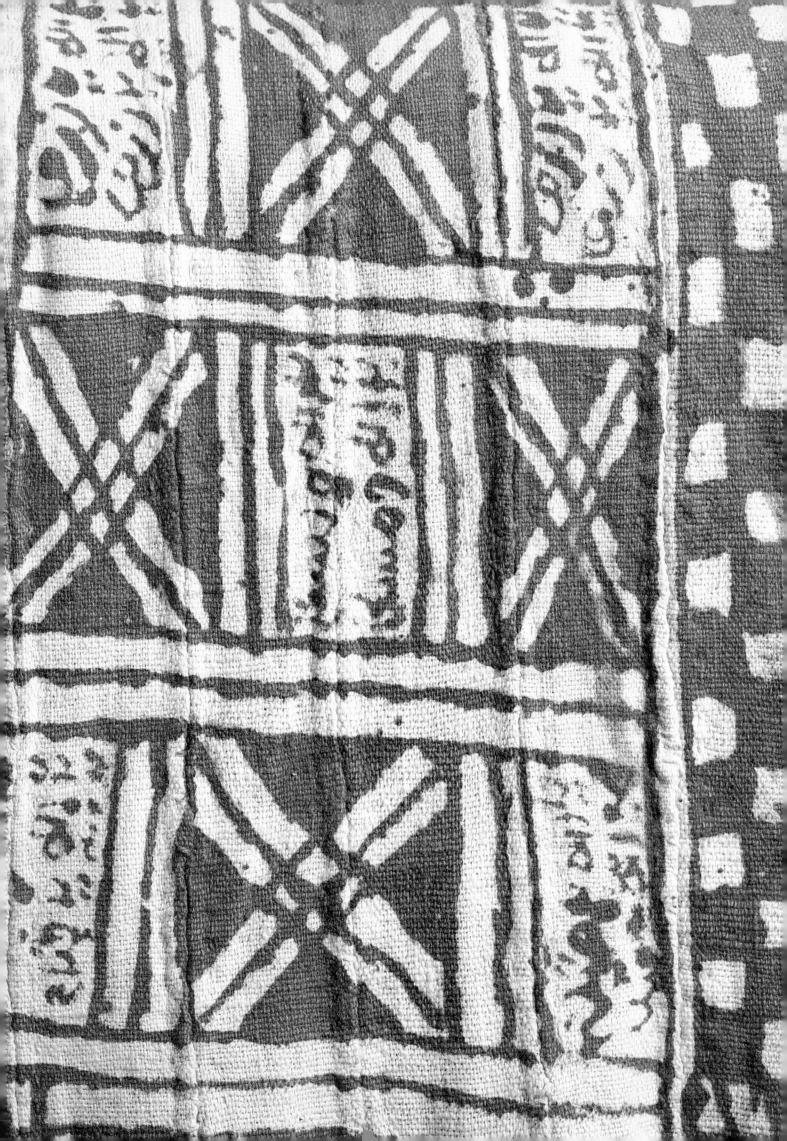

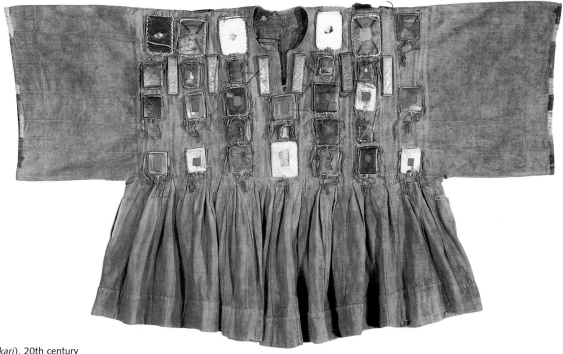

20
War shirt and belt (*batakari*), 20th century
Ghana; probably Asante
Cotton, leather, iron, fur, wool, copper;
35 ⅝ x 60 in. (shirt); 2 ½ x 57 in. (belt)

The Newark Museum, Purchase 1986 Thomas L. Raymond
Bequest Fund, 86.22a,b

geometric patterns. The pigment itself is believed to be charged with spiritual power, requiring the female artists that make *bògòlanfini* to expertly navigate the inherent dangers of its production.[49] Today, these shirts are generally worn for ceremonial occasions. A contemporary example (cat. 38), made in 1993 by Nakunte Diarra, exemplifies the clarity of design, complex patterns, and symmetrical layout that has earned this artist widespread recognition.[50]

A related form of dress is the amulet-laden war shirt, or *batakari*. Worn by men as ceremonial dress throughout western Africa, they also offer protection in the form of written prayers. In these garments, however, the prayers texts are hidden from sight, encased in pouches made of leather, fur, or fiber and occasionally adorned with metal. Originating among Islamic Mande-speaking communities, the use of war shirts spread southward and was documented among the Akan in Ghana as early as 1819.[51] The brown-dyed, strip-woven *batakari* in this exhibition (pl. 20; cat. 39), probably of Asante origin, has leather amulets as well as metal charms attached as protective elements.

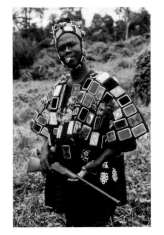

Paramount chief Odeneho Oduro Numapau II, the Omanhene (paramount chief) of the Asante state of Asumegya, in his *batakari kese* (great war-shirt), Asumegya, Ghana. Photograph by Doran Ross, 1976.

Among the Yoruba of Nigeria, diviners and priests adorn themselves with beads, which have great spiritual significance in addition to their association with royalty. As Henry Drewal and John Mason explain, "Coloring and covering the body in beads is healing and empowering. Colorful beads are *oògùn* (medicines) that act upon worldly and otherworldly forces."[52] The aesthetic brilliance of Yoruba ritual regalia, with its range of hues and myriad designs, is also deeply symbolic, marking the breadth and depth of spiritual knowledge required by religious specialists.[53] A beaded tunic worn by a Shango priest (pl. 21; cat. 40) features designs on the back representing the critical implements of office, a ritual gourd rattle (*shere Shango*) and a dance wand (*oshe Shango*).[54] Beaded necklaces worn by diviners (cat. 41), known as *òdìgbà Ifà*, have two pouches filled with empowering substances. The pouches are positioned in front of the chest and at the nape of the neck, places on the body that are especially vulnerable and in need of protection.

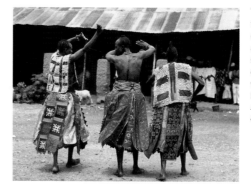

Three Yoruba priests of the thundergod Sàngó dance wearing elaborately appliqéd and paneled skirts with red serrated edges and tunics beaded with cowrie shells, Oyo, Nigeria. Photograph by Henry John Drewal, 1970 (EEPA no. A1992-028-01539).

In South Africa, beadwork ensembles had an important religious function among Xhosa-speaking peoples and, until the late twentieth century, were worn by all members of society on ceremonial occasions to contact and honor the ancestors. Made solely by women, the heaviness of layers of beadwork gave the wearer

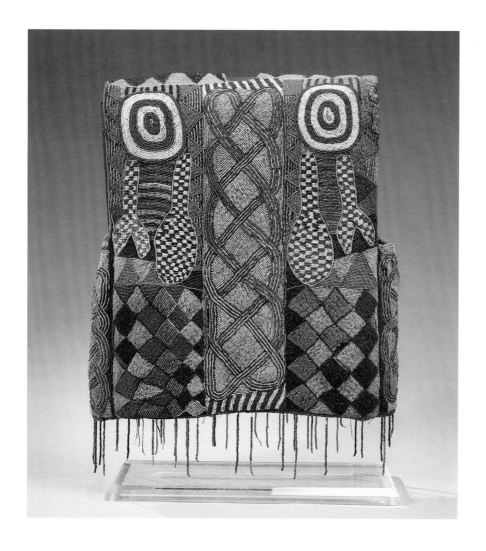

21
Tunic of a Shango priest, 20th century (back)
Nigeria; Yoruba
Cotton, beads, leather; 22 ½ x 18 ½ x 4 ½ in.

Collection Drs. Daniel and Marian Malcolm

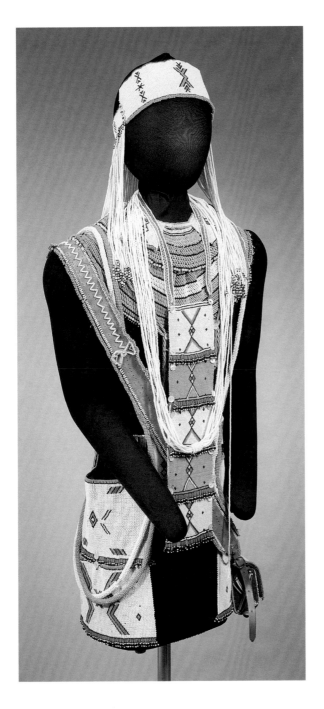

22

Ceremonial ensemble, mid-20th century
South Africa; Xhosa (Ngqika)
Beads, leather, fiber, buttons, cotton blanket;
varied dimensions

The Newark Museum, Purchase 2004 The Member's Fund,
2004.3.1.1-12

a sense of bearing the symbolic weight of the ancestors.[55] The ceremonial dress of an established Xhosa-speaking man constitutes an impressive array of beadwork, far surpassing that of his wife. In this mid-twentieth century ensemble from the Ngqika region (pl. 22; cat. 42), the most ritually significant item is the ceremonial necklace (isidanga) made of multiple strands of white beads, a color associated with purity, meditation, and supernatural clarity.[56] By the 1970s, traditional Xhosa dress was generally out of fashion, although beadwork regalia maintains its ritual relevance among some Xhosa today. In a 2000 interview, the CEO of the Xhosa Royal Council, Zolani Mkiva, described his ceremonial beadwork as a "telephone wire" connecting him with his ancestors.[57]

INNOVATION AND IDENTITY

As recent scholarship has emphasized, African dress is dynamic and evolving, with specific local histories that impact both form and meaning.[58] Almost all of the examples of men's attire featured in this exhibition demonstrate some aspect of cross-cultural influence or aesthetic inventiveness, proving that novelty is not new. Some forms of dress, however, combine elements considered traditional with those signifying modernity in innovative ways that forge a distinctive, and powerful, identity. New materials and types of clothing often serve as a creative stimulus for the transformation of local dress into novel forms of aesthetic expression, while traditional forms of dress may find new patrons or different contexts of use.

The multipiece beadwork ensemble of a Zulu man from the Msinga region in South Africa (pl. 23; cat. 43) reflects a distinct style that evolved in the period between 1930 and 1960, when clans of the Msinga region began to blend and adapt their characteristic beadwork styles and colors to reflect regional, rather than strictly clan, identity.[59] This outfit features beadwork in the Isilomi style originally associated with the Mabaso clan (a sequence of navy, turquoise, green, white, red, and black), as well as the similar Isiphalafini style (which omits turquoise). The ensemble includes traditional items, such as beaded "love token" necklaces (isijumba) of duiker hoofs and horns and a fur pelt rear apron (ibheshu). Other elements suggest the wearer's worldliness and individual sense of style. The armbands, for example, are decorated with metal chains and bicycle reflectors, and the beaded vest is of Western manufacture. Unlike women, who wear beadwork finery more frequently, men reserve such outfits for ceremonial occasions, making their visual impact all the more powerful.

A South African rickshaw driver's outfit from the 1980s (cat. 44) transforms visual elements of traditional Zulu warrior dress into a flamboyant display of extreme masculinity with its dramatic horned headress and tunic with beaded panels in the form of shields. Zulu rickshaw drivers have been a popular tourist attraction along the Durban beach front since the late

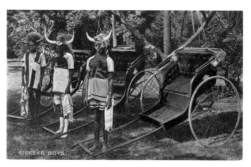

"Ricksha Boys," Zulu peoples, South Africa. Photographer unknown, c. 1920, postcard, hand-colored collotype published by A.R., Durban (No. 2). EEPA Postcard Collection SA-24-23. Eliot Elisofon Photographic Archives, National Museum of African Art, Smithsonian Institution.

nineteenth century. At first simple, their outfits have become increasingly eye-catching and outrageous since the 1950s, when rickshaw parades were first organized by the Durban Publicity Association.[60] The shield-shaped, beaded panels on this tunic have a red, green, black, and white color combination associated with the Nongoma region, the seat of the Zulu kingdom and center of power. The soaring headdress is a visual tour-de-force with dramatic woven adornments of colorful imported yarn anchored by curved ox horns painted with geometric patterns.

In Niger, Wodaabe men strive to distinguish themselves to female onlookers during Gerewol, a week-long ceremony celebrating male beauty. A man's dress is a critical component of the competition. This 1980s dance outfit (pl. 24; cat. 45) is in the form of a long, indigo-dyed tunic with elaborate chain-

23

Man's ensemble, 1950s-1960s
South Africa; Zulu (Msinga region)
Glass beads, plastic beads, brass beads, wood, string, duiker
hoofs and horn, lucite, metal chains, bicycle reflectors, fur,
chrome tacks; varied dimensions

The Newark Museum, Purchase 2005 The Member's Fund, 2005.8.1.1-14

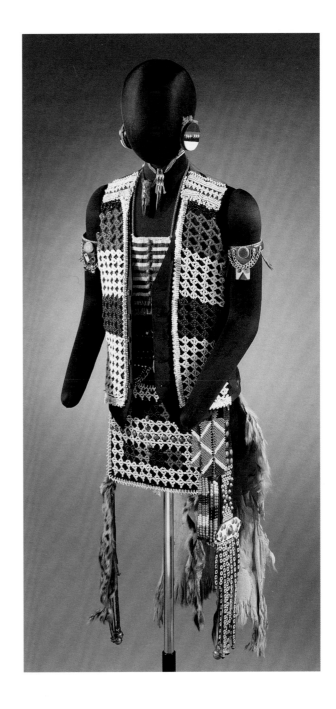

stitched embroidery in green, orange, red, yellow, and pale blue. The incorporation of new ornaments,

such as the row of shiny safety pins embellishing the front of this tunic, provides the element of flash

needed to attract attention. The use of such items, prized as imports, also demonstrates that concepts of

luxury and the exotic are culturally relative.

Embroidered tunics worn by Malian men incorporate traditional designs and nationalist symbols

with pop culture references often startling to Western eyes (cats. 46-48). According to Bernhard Gardi,

many of these tunics are made by young Malian men who have traveled south to urban centers in Ghana

for work.[61] They are worn by these migrant workers to signal their cosmopolitanism as they return from a

bustling metropolis to their rural home villages in Mali, where they are known as "Ghana boys" (*kamalen*

24
Dance ensemble, 1980s (detail: right)
Niger; Wodaabe
Cotton, leather, metal, fur, cowries, goat hair, beads, yarn,
buttons; overall h. 55 in. (varied dimensions)

The Newark Museum, Purchase 1984 The Member's Fund, 84.143a,b,
84.155, 84.164, 84.172a,b, 84.173, 84.174a,b, 84.183

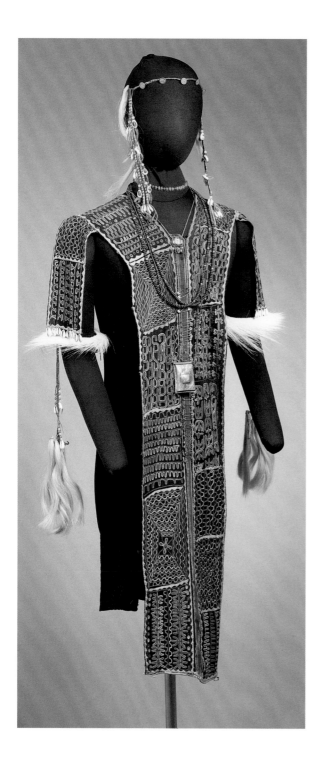

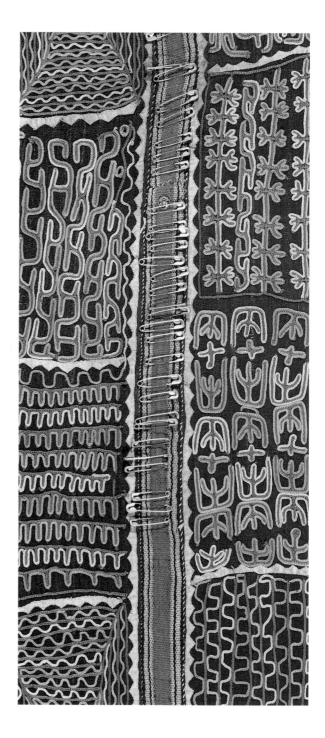

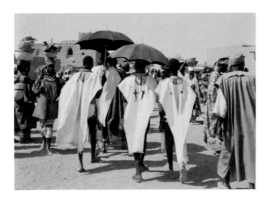

bani in Bamana). The designs on one of these tunics (pl. 25; cat. 46), embroidered with multicolored threads, combine seemingly traditional geometric motifs with icons of modernity in the form of a stop light and cigarette-smoking men on motorcycles.

The elaborate robes of Alou Traoré are simultaneously contemporary and distinctly Malian in form, and represent a recent departure from tradition-based dress, such as the hunter's tunic in this exhibition.[62] As a child, Traoré learned the technique of making *bògòlanfini*, traditionally the province of female artists, and began creating *bògòlan* clothing in the early 1990s. The man's robe here (pl. 26; cat. 49) is typical of his work, which is distinguished by its labor-intensive technique of stenciling interlocking patterns in multiple colors using different mineral

25

Tunic, ca. 1990s (back)
Djenne, Mali; Bozo or Fulani
Cotton, embroidery floss; 45 x 25 in.

The Newark Museum, Gift of Joseph Knopfelmacher 1997, 97.22.1

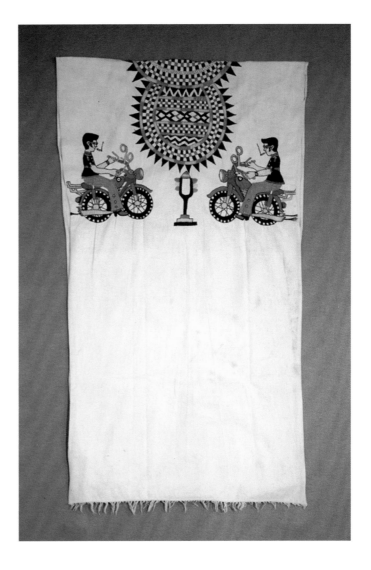

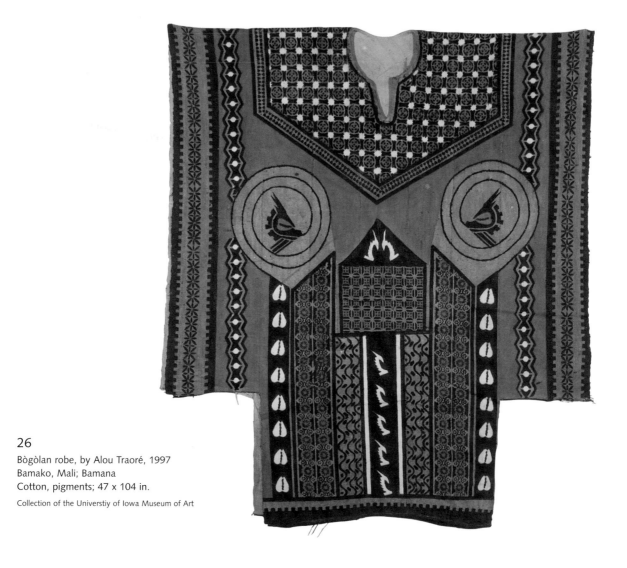

26
Bògòlan robe, by Alou Traoré, 1997
Bamako, Mali; Bamana
Cotton, pigments; 47 x 104 in.
Collection of the Universtiy of Iowa Museum of Art

and vegetal dyes. The designs on his cloth transform tradition, as they reference motifs that have come to be associated with Malian nationalism, such as Bamana *ci wara* headdresses, cowrie shells, and dancers, instead of Bamana designs with local meanings.[63] Produced mostly on commission, Traoré's clothing enjoys popularity among urban clients, particularly musicians and other entertainers, in Bamako and elsewhere.[64]

Today, with more African immigrants arriving in the United States each year than did enslaved immigrants at the height of the slave trade, a new African diaspora is emerging in both cities and sub-urbs, impacting the realm of fashion. In Newark, New Jersey, Guinea-born tailor Amadou Diallo runs a thriving dress shop that is patronized by fellow West Africans, African Americans, and others drawn to his vibrant clothing and skills as a tailor. Imported fabrics arrive from West Africa with frequency and posters of popular urban styles adorn the walls of the shop, allowing recent immigrants to keep up with the fashions of home. The traditional-style men's wedding ensemble with gold thread embroidery (cat. 50) in this exhibition is described by Diallo as one that might be worn by a wealthy man in either Conakry, the capital of Guinea, or at a celebration in New Jersey. It serves as a visual reminder that African dress transcends the continent and today, more than ever, has a global impact.[65]

NOTES

1. Eliot Elisofon trip notes, Nigeria essay captions. Rolls K80 (frames 25 to end), K81 (frames 21 to end), K82 (entire roll), November 19, 1959. Eliot Elisofon Photographic Archives, National Museum of African Art, Smithsonian Institution.

2. Henry Drewal, in Drewal and John Mason, *Beads Body and Soul: Art and Light in the Yoruba Universe* (Los Angeles: UCLA Fowler Museum of Cultural History, 1998), 58.

3. Of course, there are many important exceptions to this generality. For example, a recent publication, edited by Jean Allman, prompts a reconsideration of "our ideas of both 'the public' and 'the political' as predominantly male spaces...its focus on bodily praxis renders women's political praxis visible and sharply focused in stories of emancipation and citizenship and of nation-building and nationalism." See Jean Allman, ed., *Fashioning Africa: Power and the Politics of Dress* (Bloomington: Indiana University Press, 2004), 5.

4. Although this exhibition focuses on garments and accessories, dress—in its broadest definition—may include modifications to the body itself, such as tattoos and hairstyles. See Ruth Barnes and Joanne Eicher, eds. *Dress and Gender: Making and Meaning in Cultural Contexts* (Providence: Berg, 1992).

5. Fred Davis, *Fashion, Culture and Identity* (Chicago and London: The University of Chicago Press, 1992), 11.

6. Barnes and Eicher, 1.

7. Allman, 1.

8. Frieda Sorber, "Siroua Costumes," in Niloo Imami Paydar and Ivo Grammet, eds., *The Fabric of Moroccan Life* (Indianapolis: Indianapolis Museum of Art, 2002), 251.

9. Ibid., 252.

10. This distinctive form of African men's clothing has been the subject of an exhibition at the Museum der Kulturen Basel in 2000 and an accompanying catalogue, edited by Bernhard Gardi, which represents a rich addition to the study of African dress. See Bernhard Gardi, *Le boubou—c'est chic: Les boubous du Mali et d'autres pays de l'Afrique de l'Ouest*, Basel: Museum der Kuturen Basel/ Christoph Merian, 2002. Second edition.

11. Colleen E. Kriger, "Textile Production and Gender in the Sokoto Caliphate," *The Journal of African History*, vol. 34, no. 3 (1993), 389.

12. Colleen E. Kriger, *Cloth in West African History*, Lanham, MD: AltaMira Press, forthcoming.

13. David Heathcote, "A Hausa Charm Gown," *Man, New Series*, vol. 9, no. 4 (1974), 623.

14. Kriger, 390.

15. Judith Perani and Norma H. Wolff, *Cloth, Dress and Art Patronage in Africa* (Oxford and New York: Berg, 1999), 121.

16. David Heathcote, "Hausa Embroidered Dress," *African Arts*, vol. 5, no. 2 (1972), 15. In this article, Heathcote notes changes in the last two decades, with men wearing lighter and narrower gowns with less embroidery, and older men preferring larger amounts of embroidered cloth.

17. Perani and Wolff, 141.

18. See Elisha Renne's "From Khaki to *Agbada*: Dress and Political Transition in Nigeria," in Allman, 125-43.

19. Venice Lamb and Judy Holmes, *Nigerian Weaving* (Lagos: Shell Petroleum Development Company of Nigeria Ltd., 1980), 55.

20. Ibid, 52.

21. The text has been transcribed as *Lelelele laiye olowo fara molowo*, a variant of the Yoruba proverb *Afefe laye olowo fara molowo*, translated as, "The wind is in the world, the rich keep together with the rich." The translation was provided by Dr. Akin Oyetade, School of Oriental and African Studies, London, according to Duncan Clarke, letter to Anne Spencer, January 21, 1995. Object Records, The Newark Museum.

22. Margaret Carey, *Beads and Beadwork of East and South Africa* (Shire Ethnography Publications, 1986), 18-19.

23. Daniel P. Biebuyck, "Lega Dress as Cultural Artifact," *African Arts*, vol. 15, no. 3 (1982), 61-62.

24. Ibid., 62.

25. Elisabeth L. Cameron, "Lega Hats: Hierarchy and Status," in Mary Jo Arnoldi and Christine Kreamer, eds., *Crowning Achievements: African Arts of Dressing the Head* (Los Angeles: UCLA Fowler Museum of Cultural History, 1995), 155.

26. Perani and Wolff, 90.

27. Ibid., 90.

28. Suzanne Blier, *The Royal Arts of Africa* (New York: Abrams, 1998), 231.

29. Doran Ross, *Gold of the Akan from the Glassell Collection* (Houston: Museum of Fine Arts, 2002), 133.

30. Ibid., 140, 143.

31. Doran Ross, personal communication, July 2005.

32. Drewal and Mason, 218.

33. Transcription by Nii Quarcoopome according to Bernard Wagner, personal communication, June 2005.

34. Drewal and Mason, 217-18.

35. Arnoldi and Kreamer, 47.

36. Blier, 120.

37. Alexandre Adande, *Les Récades des Rois du Dahomey* (Dakar: IFAN – Institut Français D'Afrique Noire, 1962), 77.

38. Ibid., 17.

39. Silvia Forni, personal communication, July 2005.

40. Ibid. The association of this ensemble with kingly power is also suggested by its formal resemblance to the quill-studded masquerade costumes of Ngirrih, a secret society of princes and other members of the royal family recently introduced in the kingdom of Oku. See Hans-Joachim Koloss, *World-View and Society in Oku (Cameroon)* (Berlin: Von Dietrich Reimer, 2000), 266-72. Father Hermann Gufler, a longtime resident of Cameroon, has also documented the "Princes society" masquerade and noted the association of porcupine quills with the chief and royal family. Gufler, personal communication, August 2005.

41. Arnoldi and Kreamer, 107, 113.

42. Tamara Northern, *The Art of Cameroon* (Washington, D.C.: Smithsonian Institution Press, 1984), 54.

43. Alice Euretta Horner, "The Assumption of Tradition: Creating, Collecting, and Conserving Cultural Artifacts in the Cameroon Grassfields" (Ph.D. dissertation, Department of Anthropology, University of California, Berkeley, 1990), 134.

44. Ibid., 140, 159.

45. Christopher Spring and Julie Hudson, *North African Textiles* (Washington, D.C.: Smithsonian Institution Press, 1995), 104.

46. John Picton and John Mack, *African Textiles* (New York: Harper & Row, 1989), 173.

47. Rene A. Bravmann, *African Islam* (Washington, D.C.: Smithsonian Institution Press, 1983), 26-27.

48. See Patrick McNaughton, "The Shirts That Mande Hunters Wear," *African Arts*, vol. 15, no. 3 (1982), 54-58, 91.

49. Victoria L. Rovine, *Bogolan: Shaping Culture through Cloth in Contemporary Mali* (Washington, D.C.: Smithsonian Instititution Press, 2001), 25.

50. See especially Tavy Aherne, *Nakunte Diarra: Bògòlanfini Artist of the Beledougou* (Bloomington: Indiana University Art Museum, 1992).

51. Herbert M. Cole and Doran H. Ross, *The Arts of Ghana* (Los Angeles: Museum of Cultural History, UCLA, 1977), 18.

52. Drewal and Mason, 17.

53. Drewal and Mason, 228.

54. Henry Drewal, personal communication, March 2005.

55. Gary van Wyk, "Illuminated Signs: Style and Meaning in the Beadwork of the Xhosa- and Zulu-speaking Peoples," *African Arts*, vol. 36, no. 3 (2003), 24.

56. Ibid., 18-19.

57. As noted by Lisa Brittan. Ibid., 24.

58. Most recently, a 2004 edited publication by Jean Allman foregrounds African histories in dismantling the established binary of tradition versus modernity. An earlier work edited by Hildi Hendrickson, *Clothing and Difference: Embodied Identities in Colonial and Post-Colonial Africa* (Durham: Duke University Press, 1996) challenges the underlying premise of the Western world that associates fashion exclusively with modernity.

59. Van Wyk, 28. See also Frank Jolles, "Traditional Beadwork of the Msinga Area," *African Arts*, vol. 26, no. 1 (1993), 42-56, 101-02.

60. Craig Jacobs, "The Shame and the Glory," *Sunday Times*, Johannesburg, South Africa, November 19, 2000.

61. Gardi, 27.

62. Victoria Rovine, "Fashionable Traditions: The Globalization of an African Textile," in Allman, 196.

63. Rovine, 127.

64. Ibid.

65. An insightful study of the shifting markets for and meanings of African and African-style textiles and dress may be found in Leslie W. Rabine's *The Global Circulation of African Fashion* (New York: Berg, 2002).

SELECT BIBLIOGRAPHY

Compiled by Harriet Walker

Adande, Alexandre. *Les Recades des Rois du Dahomey*. Dakar: Institut Francais D'Afrique Noire, 1962.

Aherne, Tavy D. *Nakunte Diarra: Bògòlanfini Artist of the Beledougou*. Bloomington: Indiana University Art Museum, 1992.

Allman, Jean Marie. *Fashioning Africa: Power and the Politics of Dress*. Bloomington: Indiana University Press, 2004.

Arnoldi, Mary Jo, and Christine Kreamer. *Crowning Achievements: African Arts of Dressing the Head*. Los Angeles: UCLA Fowler Museum of Cultural History, 1995.

Barnes, Ruth, and Joanne Eicher (eds). *Dress and Gender: Making and Meaning in Cultural Contexts*. Providence, RI: Berg, 1992.

Beckwith, Carol (photographs) and Marion Van Offelen (text). *Nomads of Niger*. New York: Abrams, 1983.

Bedford, Emma (ed). *Ezakwantu: Beadwork from the Eastern Cape*. Cape Town: South African National Gallery, 1993.

Biebuyck, Daniel. "Lega Dress as Cultural Artifact," *African Arts*, vol. 15, no. 3 (1982): 59-65, 92.

Blier, Suzanne. *The Royal Arts of Africa*. New York: Abrams, 1998.

Bourgeois, Arthur P. "Yaka and Suku Leadership Headgear," *African Arts*, vol. 15, no. 3 (1982): 30-35, 92.

Boyer, Ruth. "Yoruba Cloths with Regal Names," *African Arts*, vol. 16, no. 2 (1983): 42-45, 98.

Bravmann, Rene A. *African Islam*. Washington, D.C.: Smithsonian Institution Press, 1983.

Broster, Joan, and Alice Mertens. *African Elegance*. Capetown/New York: Purnell and Sons, 1973.

Carey, Margaret. *Beads and Beadwork of East and South Africa*. London: Shire Ethnography Publications, 1986.

Clarke, Duncan. *The Art of African Textiles*. San Diego: Thunder Bay Press, 1997.

Cole, Herbert, and Doran Ross. *The Arts of Ghana*. Los Angeles: Museum of Cultural History, UCLA, 1977.

Cordwell, Justine. "The Art and Aesthetics of the Yoruba," *African Arts*, vol. 16, no. 2 (1983): 56-59, 92-94, 100.

Davis, Fred. *Fashion, Culture and Identity*. Chicago/London: University of Chicago Press, 1992.

De Negri, Eve. "Yoruba Men's Costume," *Nigeria Magazine* 73 (1962): 4-12.

Drewal, Henry, and John Mason. *Beads Body and Soul: Art and Light in the Yoruba Universe*. Los Angeles: UCLA Fowler Museum of Cultural History, 1998.

Drewal, Margaret Thompson. "Art and Trance among Yoruba Shango Devotees," *African Arts*, vol. 20, no. 1 (1986): 60-67, 98-99.

Eicher, Joanne. *African Dress: A Select and Annotated Bibliography of Sub-Saharan Countries*. East Lansing: Michigan State University, 1969.

——. "Africa. Dress," in *The Dictionary of Art*, ed. Jane Turner. New York: Grove Dictionaries, 1996.

Elliott, Aubrey. *Magic World of the Xhosa*. New York: Scribner, 1970.

Frank, Barbara. *Mande Potters and Leather Workers: Art and Heritage in West Africa*. Washington, D.C.: Smithsonian Institution Press, 1998.

Fraser, Douglas, and Herbert M. Cole (eds). *African Art and Leadership*. Madison: University of Wisconsin Press, 1972.

Gardi, Bernhard. *Le boubou—c'est chic: Les boubous du Mali et d'autres pays de l'Afrique de l'Ouest*. 2nd edition. Basel: Museum der Kulturen Basel/Christoph Merian, 2002.

Gebauer, Paul. *Art of Cameroon*: Portland, OR: Portland Art Museum, 1979.

Hansen, Karen Tranberg. "The World in Dress: Anthropological Perspectives on Clothing, Fashion, and Culture," *Annual Review of Anthropology*, vol. 33 (October 2004): 369-92.

Heathcote, David. "Hausa Embroidered Dress," *African Arts*, vol. 5, no. 2 (1972): 12-19, 82, 84.

Heathcote, David. "A Hausa Embroiderer of Katsina," *Nigerian Field*, vol. 37, no. 3 (1972): 123-31.

Heathcote, David. "Insight into a Creative Process: A Rare Collection of Embroidery Drawings from Kano," *Savana*, vol. 1, no. 2 (1972): 165-74.

Heathcote, David. "A Hausa Charm Gown," *Man, New Series*, vol. 9, no. 4 (1974): 620-24.

Hendrickson, Hildi, ed. *Clothing and Difference: Embodied Identities in Colonial and Post-Colonial Africa*. Durham, NC: Duke University Press, 1996.

Herskovits, Melville. *Dahomey: An Ancient West African Kingdom*. New York: J.J. Augustin, 1938.

Horner, Alice. *Assumption of Tradition: Creating, Collecting, and Conserving Cultural Artifacts in the Cameroon Grassfields*. Ph.D. dissertation, Department of Anthropology, University of California, Berkeley, 1990.

Jolles, Frank. "Traditional Zulu Beadwork of the Msinga Arts," *African Arts*, vol. 26, no. 1 (1993): 42-56, 101-02.

Koloss, Hans-Joachim. *World-View and Society in Oku (Cameroon)*. Berlin: Von Dietrich Reimer, 2000.

Kriger, Colleen. "Robes of the Sokoto Caliphate," *African Arts*, vol. 21, no. 3 (1988): 52-57, 78-79, 85-86.

——. "Textile Production and Gender in the Sokoto Caliphate," *Journal of African History*, vol. 34, no. 3 (1993): 361-401.

Lamb, Venice. *West African Weaving*. London: Duckworth and Co., 1975.

——. *Au Cameroun: Weaving—Tissage*. Hertingfordbury: Roxford Books, 1981.

Lamb, Venice, and Judy Holmes. *Nigerian Weaving*. Lagos: Shell Petroleum Development Company of Nigeria, 1980.

McNaughton, Patrick R. "The Shirts that Mande Hunters Wear," *African Arts*, vol. 15, no. 3 (1982): 54-58, 91.

Morris, Jean, and Eleanor Preston-Whyte. *Speaking with Beads: Zulu Arts from Southern Africa*. New York: Thames and Hudson, 1994.

Nooter, Nancy Ingram. "Africa. Regalia," in *The Dictionary of Art*, ed. Jane Turner. New York: Grove's Dictionaries, 1996.

Northern, Tamara. *The Art of Cameroon*. Washington, D.C.: Smithsonian Institution Press, 1984.

Paydar, Niloo, and Ivo Grammet (eds.). *The Fabric of Moroccan Life*. Indianapolis, IN: Indianapolis Museum of Art, 2002.

Pemberton, John, Rowland Abiodun, and Ulli Beier. *Cloth Only Wears to Shreds: Yoruba Textiles and Photographs from the Beier Collection*. Amherst, MA: Mead Art Museum, Amherst College, 2004.

Perani, Judith. "Patronage and Nupe Craft Industries," *African Arts*, vol. 13, no. 3 (1980): 71-75, 92.

Perani, Judith, and Norma H. Wolff. "Embroidered Gown and Equestrian Ensembles of the Kano Aristocracy," *African Arts,* vol. 25, no. 3 (1992): 70-81, 102-04.

——. *Cloth, Dress, and Art Patronage in Africa.* Oxford/New York: Berg, 1999.

Picton, John, and John Mack. *African Textiles.* New York: Harper and Row, 1989.

——. *The Art of African Textiles: Technology, Tradition, and Lurex.* London: Barbican Art Gallery; Lund Humphries Publishers, 1995.

Pique, Francesca, and Leslie Rainer. *Palace Sculptures of Abomey: History Told on Walls.* Los Angeles: Getty Conservation Institute, 1999.

Rabine, Leslie W. *The Global Circulation of African Fashion.* New York: Berg, 2002.

Renne, Elisha. "The Thierry Collection of Hausa Artifacts at the Field Museum," *African Arts,* vol. 19, no. 4 (1986): 54-59, 85.

Ross, Doran. *Wrapped in Pride: Ghanaian Kente and African American Identity.* Los Angeles: UCLA Fowler Museum of Cultural History, 1998.

——. *Gold of the Akan from the Glassell Collection.* Houston: Museum of Fine Arts, Houston, 2002.

Rovine, Victoria. *Bogolan: Shaping Culture through Cloth in Contemporary Mali.* Washington, D.C.: Smithsonian Institution Press, 2001.

Schaedler, Karl-Ferdinand. *Weaving in Africa South of the Sahara.* Munchen: Panterra-Verlag, 1987.

Sieber, Roy. *African Textiles and Decorative Arts.* New York: Museum of Modern Art, 1972.

Spring, Christopher, and Julie Hudson. *North African Textiles.* Washington, D.C.: Smithsonian Institution Press, 1995.

Thieme, Otto C., and Joanne Eicher. "African Dress: Form, Action, Meaning," *African Journal,* vol. 14, nos. 2-3 (1983): 115-38.

Tyrrell, Barbara. *Tribal Peoples of Southern Africa.* Cape Town: Books of Africa, 1968.

Van Wyk, Gary. "Illuminated Signs: Style and Meaning in the Beadwork of the Xhosa and Zulu-speaking Peoples," *African Arts,* vol. 36, no. 3 (2003): 12-33, 93-94.

CHECKLIST OF THE EXHIBITION

*illustrated in catalogue

INTRODUCTION

1* Ceremonial robe of the Déjì of Akure,
late 19th – early 20th century
Akure, Ekiti region, Nigeria; Yoruba
Cotton, velvet, beads; 50 x 104 ½ in.
The Newark Museum, Purchase 1993 John
J. O'Neil Bequest Fund & The Member's
Fund, 93.268

STYLE AND STATUS

2* Cloak (akhnif), late 19th – early 20th century
Sus region, Morocco; Ait Ouaouzguite
Wool; 63 x 71 ½ in.
The Newark Museum, Purchase 1927,
The J. Ackerman Coles Collection, 27.105

3* Robe (riga), 1920s
Zaria, Nigeria; Hausa
Cotton, wool; 57 x 103 in.
The Newark Museum, Purchase 1929,
29.673

4 Drawstring trousers (wando mai surfani),
early to mid-20th century
Nigeria; Hausa
Cotton; 44 x 184 in.
The Newark Museum, Purchase 1985
O.W. Caspersen Bequest Fund, 85.361

5 Riding boots, late 19th – early 20th century
Zaria, Nigeria; Hausa
Leather, pigment; 32 ½ x 9 x 9 ¾ in. (a);
32 ½ x 9 ¾ x 10 in. (b)
The Newark Museum, Purchase 1928,
28.1913a,b

6 Prestige staff (mashi), possibly owned by
the Emir of Zaria, before 1928
Zaria, Nigeria; Hausa
Iron, brass; 59 ½ x 1 ¾ x 1 ⅝ in.
The Newark Museum, Purchase 1928,
28.1912

7* Robe (agbada), early 20th century
Oyo, Nigeria; Yoruba
Silk, cotton; 49 x 97 in.
The Newark Museum, Purchase 1986 The
Member's Fund, 86.240

8 Robe (agbada), early to mid-20th century
Nigeria; Yoruba
Cotton; 53 ½ x 104 in.
The Newark Museum, Gift of Mrs. Harrison
F. Durand 1974, 74.105

9* Robe (dandogo), mid-20th century
Nigeria; Yoruba
Cotton; 46 ½ x 109 in.
The Newark Museum, Purchase 1983,
Wallace M. Scudder Bequest Fund, 83.102

10* Man's corset, second half of the 20th century
Sudan; Dinka
Beads, fiber, leather; 30 x 14 ½ in.
The Newark Museum, Purchase 2005 The
Member's Fund, 2005.14

11* Headdress (sawamazembe), 20th century
Democratic Republic of the Congo; Lega
Fiber, shells, buttons, seed pods;
16 ¾ x 10 in.
Private Collection

12 Headdress (mukuba wa bifungo),
20th century
Democratic Republic of the Congo; Lega
Beads, fiber, shells, buttons, elephant tail,
seed pods; 14 ½ x 10 ½ in.
Private Collection

13 Headdress, 20th century
Democratic Republic of the Congo; Lega
Pangolin scales, fiber, buttons, shells;
17 x 9 ½ in.
Private Collection

FIT FOR A KING

14 Royal man's skirt
Democratic Republic of the Congo; Kuba
Raffia; 32 ½ x 293 ½ in.
The Newark Museum, Purchase 1993
Thomas L Raymond Bequest Fund &
Franklin Conklin Jr. Memorial Fund, 93.81

15* Ceremonial shirt and cap worn by King
Mbop Mabiine maKyeen, before 1969
Democratic Republic of the Congo; Kuba
Raffia, cowries, fur, copper, beads, feathers;
28 x 61 in. (shirt); 4 ¾ x 6 ½ in. (cap);
The Newark Museum, Purchase 1982
Wallace M. Scudder Bequest Fund, 82.195a,b

16 Disk pendant (akrafokonmu), 20th century
Ghana; Asante
Wood, gold leaf; 4 ⅝ x 4 ⅝ x 1 ⅞ in.
The Newark Museum, Gift of Dr. and Mrs.
Eugene Becker, 1986, 86.251

17* Disk pendant (akrafokonmu), 20th century
Ghana; Asante
Cast gold; 4 x 4 x 1 in.
The Newark Museum, Purchase 1987
William M. Scudder Bequest Fund, 87.35

18 Bracelet (benkum benfra), 20th century
Ghana; Asante
Wood, gold leaf; 5 ½ x 4 ⅜ x 2 in.
The Newark Museum, Gift of Dr. and Mrs.
Eugene Becker, 1986 86.252A-C

19 Sandals (mpaboa), 20th century
Ghana; Asante
Leather, velvet, gold leaf, cowrie shells;
11 ⅝ x 6 in. (a); 11 ¾ x 6 in. (b)
The Newark Museum, Purchase 1985
Wallace M. Scudder Bequest Fund and
Sophronia Anderson Bequest Fund,
85.365a,b

20* Crown, 20th century
Ghana; Asante
Wood, velvet, cotton, gold leaf;
8 ¾ x 8 x 8 in.
The Newark Museum, Purchase 1986
Eleanor S. Upton Bequest Fund, 86.247

21 Kente wrapper, ca. 1930
Ghana; Asante
Rayon; 112 x 152 in.
The Newark Museum, Gift of Mr. & Mrs.
William U. Wright 1985, 85.366

22* "Cloth of the great" (akunitan), 1957-66
Ghana; Akan
Wool, rayon thread; 75 ½ x 115 ½ in.
The Newark Museum, Purchase 2005 The
Membership Endowment Fund, 2005.2

23 Crown (adénlá), 20th century
Nigeria; Yoruba
Fabric, glass beads, thread; 54 ½ x 30 in.
Collection Dr. and Mrs. Bernard Wagner

24* Slippers (bàtà ilèkè), 20th century
Efon-Alaye, Ekiti region, Nigeria; Yoruba
Beads, leather, thread; 10 x 3 ½ in.
Collection Dr. and Mrs. Bernard Wagner

25* Foot cushion (timùtimù), 20th century
Efon-Alaye, Ekiti region, Nigeria; Yoruba
Beads, leather; 7 x 19 ¼ in.
Collection Dr. and Mrs. Bernard Wagner

26 Crown (oríkògbòfó), 20th century
Nigeria; Yoruba
Raffia, canvas, glass beads; 28 x 7 in.
Collection Dr. and Mrs. Bernard Wagner

27* Ensemble of a royal or noble,
late 19th century
Republic of Benin; Fon
Cotton, silk; 34 ¼ x 27 ⁹⁄₁₆ in. (tunic);
29 ½ x 26 in. (trousers);
3 ⅛ x 6 ¹¹⁄₁₆ x 6 ¹¹⁄₁₆ in. (cap)
Brooklyn Museum, Museum Expedition
1922, Robert B. Woodward Memorial
Fund, 22.1200a-b (tunic and trousers);
22.1501 (cap)

28 Ritual staff, mid-20th century
Republic of Benin; Fon
Wood, sheet brass; 23 x 13 ¼ x 1 ½ in.
The Newark Museum, Purchase 2005
Wallace Scudder Bequest Fund, 2005.17.1

29 Royal staff, late 19th century
Republic of Benin; Fon
Wood, steel; 19 ¼ x 1 ¾ x 8 ½ in.
The Newark Museum, Purchase 1924
Walter Dormitzer Collection, 24.453

30* Ceremonial ensemble, late 20th century
Grassfields region, Cameroon
Cotton, leather, porcupine quills;
38 ½ x 22 ½ in. (tunic); 16 x 9 x 9 in. (hat)
Private Collection

31* Headdress, 20th century
Cameroon; Bamileke
Feathers, fiber; 20 x 30 ¼ x 30 ¼ in. (open)
The Newark Museum, Purchase 1980
Harry E. Saulter Bequest Fund, 80.35

32* Headdress, 20th century
Cameroon; Bamileke
Feathers, fiber; 13 ¼ x 8 x 8 in. (closed)
The Newark Museum, Purchase 1980
C.W. Caspersen Bequest Fund, 80.36

33* Ceremonial ensemble, 1992
Cameroon; Bafut
Polyester, cotton; 50 x 80 ½ in. (gown);
35 x 32 in., 38 ½ x 32 in. (2-piece skirt);
10 x 10 x 10 in. (hat)
The Newark Museum, Purchase 1994
Membership Endowment Fund, 94.97a

34 Chief's headdress (botolo), 20th century
Democratic Republic of the Congo; Ekonda
Vegetable fiber, brass; 15 ¾ x 8 ¼ in.
Private collection

35 Chief's headdress (misango mayaka),
20th century
Democratic Republic of the Congo; Yaka
Beads, fiber: 6 x 17 ½ x 11 ¾ in.
Private collection

DIVINE DRESS

36* Tunic (jibbeh), c. 1881-1898
Sudan; Mahdist
Cotton, linen; 38 x 59 ¾ in.
The Newark Museum, Purchase 1924
Membership Receipts, The Albert E. Barnes
Collection, 24.301

37* Tunic, late 19th century
Togo
Cotton, pigment; 48 x w. 54 ¼ in.
The Newark Museum, Purchase 1993
Wallace M. Scudder Bequest Fund, 93.269

38 Hunter's tunic (donson dlokiw), by Nakunte
Diarra, 1992
Beledegou region, Mali; Bamana
Bògòlan pigments on strip-woven cotton;
30 x 31 in.
Collection of the University of Iowa
Museum of Art

39* War shirt and belt (batakari), 20th century
Ghana; probably Asante
Cotton, leather, iron, fur, wool, copper;
35 ⅝ x 60 in. (shirt); 2 ½ x 57 in. (belt)
The Newark Museum, Purchase 1986
Thomas L. Raymond Bequest Fund, 86.22a,b

40* Tunic and flywhisk of a Shango priest,
20th century
Nigeria; Yoruba
Cotton, beads, leather; 22 ²/₄ x 18 ½ x 4 ½ in.
(tunic); 21 ½ x 1 ⅛ x 1 ⅛ in. (flywhisk)
Collection Drs. Daniel and Marian Malcolm

41 Diviner's necklace (òdìgbà Ifá), 20th century
Nigeria; Yoruba
Cloth, glass beads, leather, string; 22 x 34 in.
Collection Dr. and Mrs. Bernard Wagner

42* Ceremonial ensemble, mid-20th century
South Africa; Xhosa (Ngqika)
Beads, leather, fiber, buttons, cotton blanket;
varied dimensions
The Newark Museum, Purchase 2004 The
Member's Fund, 2004.3.1.1-12

INNOVATION AND IDENTITY

43* Man's ensemble, 1950s-1960s
South Africa; Zulu (Msinga region)
Glass beads, plastic beads, brass beads,
wood, string, duiker hoofs and horn,
lucite, metal chains, bicycle reflectors, fur,
chrome tacks; varied dimensions
The Newark Museum, Purchase 2005 The
Member's Fund, 2005.8.1.1-14

44 Rickshaw driver's outfit, c. 1980
Durban, South Africa; Zulu (Nongoma
region)
Glass beads, horn, pigment, yarn, feathers,
mirrors, leather; 48 x 43 x 18 in. (headdress); 52 x 23 x 6 in. (tunic)
Collection Axis Gallery, New York

45* Dance ensemble, 1980s
Niger; Wodaabe
Cotton, leather, metal, fur, cowries, goat
hair, beads, yarn, buttons; overall h. 55 in.
(varied dimensions)
The Newark Museum, Purchase 1984 The
Member's Fund, 84.143a,b, 84.155, 84.164,
84.172a,b, 84.173, 84.174a,b, 84.183

46* Tunic, ca. 1990s
Djenne, Mali; Bozo or Fulani
Cotton, embroidery floss; 45 x 25 in.
The Newark Museum, Gift of Joseph
Knopfelmacher 1997, 97.22.1

47 Tunic, ca. 1990s
Djenne, Mali; Bozo or Fulani
Cotton, embroidery floss; 45 x 49 in.
The Newark Museum, Gift of Joseph
Knopfelmacher 1997, 97.22.2

48 Tunic, ca. 1990s
Djenne, Mali; Bozo or Fulani
Cotton, embroidery floss; 40 x 26 ½ in.
The Newark Museum, Gift of Joseph
Knopfelmacher 1997, 97.22.

49 Bògòlan robe, by Alou Traoré, 1997
Bamako, Mali; Bamana
Cotton, pigments; 104 x 47 in.
Collection of the Universtiy of Iowa
Museum of Art

50 Man's wedding outfit, by Amadou Diallo,
2004
Newark, New Jersey, USA; Fula
Cotton, rayon; 54 ¼ x 50 ½ in. (robe);
34 ⅛ x 61 ¾ in. (shirt); 42 ½ x 27 in. (pants)
The Newark Museum, Purchase 2004
Estate of Clara Streissquth, 2004.33.1a-c